Nurse Aide Practice Questions

Complete Test Preparation

Test Preparation Publishing
Victoria BC Canada

Copyright © 2011 by Brian Stocker. ALL RIGHTS RESERVED. No part of this book may be reproduced or transferred in any form or by any means, graphic, electronic, or mechanical, including photocopying, recording, web distribution, taping, or by any information storage retrieval system, without the written permission of the author.

Notice: Complete Test Preparation makes every reasonable effort to obtain from reliable sources accurate, complete, and timely information about the tests covered in this book. Nevertheless, changes can be made in the tests or the administration of the tests at any time and Complete Test Preparation makes no representation or warranty, either expressed or implied as to the accuracy, timeliness, or completeness of the information contained in this book. Complete Test Preparation make no representations or warranties of any kind, express or implied, about the completeness, accuracy, reliability, suitability or availability with respect to the information contained in this document for any purpose. Any reliance you place on such information is therefore strictly at your own risk.

The author(s) shall not be liable for any loss incurred as a consequence of the use and application, directly or indirectly, of any information presented in this work. Sold with the understanding, the author is not engaged in rendering professional services or advice. If advice or expert assistance is required, the services of a competent professional should be sought.

The company, product and service names used in this publication are for identification purposes only. All trademarks and registered trademarks are the property of their respective owners. Complete Test Preparation is not affiliate with any educational institution.

We strongly recommend that students check with exam providers for up-to-date information regarding test content.

ISBN-13: 978-1480127678
ISBN-10: 1480127671

Study >> Practice >> Succeed!

Complete Test Preparation

Published by
Complete Test Preparation
921 Foul Bay Rd.
Victoria BC Canada V8S 4H9
Visit us on the web at http://www.test-preparation.ca
Printed in the USA

About Complete Test Preparation

The Complete Test Preparation Team has been publishing high quality study materials since 2005. Millions of students visit our websites every year, and thousands of students, teachers and parents all over the world have purchased our teaching materials, curriculum, study guides and practice tests.

Complete Test Preparation is committed to providing students with the best study materials and practice tests available on the market. Members of our team combine years of teaching experience, with experienced writers and editors, all with advanced degrees (Masters or higher).

Team Members for this publication

Editor: Brian Stocker MA
Contributor: D. Tovander PhD.
Contributor: Dr. G. A. Stocker DDS
Contributor: D. A. Stocker M. Ed.

Study >> Practice >> Succeed!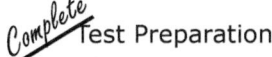

Contents

6 Getting Started

8 Practice Test Questions Set
- Quick Reference Answer Key — 27
- Answer Key with Explanations — 28

37 Practice Test Questions Set 2
- Quick Reference Answer Key — 55
- Answer Key with Explanations — 56

64 How to Prepare for a Test
- Mental Prep – Psych Yourself Up — 67

69 How to Take a Test
- How to Take a Test - The Basics — 69
- In the Test Room — 74
- Avoid Anxiety Prior to a Test — 80
- Common Test-Taking Mistakes — 82

85 Conclusion

86 Customizing and White Label Service

Getting Started

CONGRATULATIONS! By deciding to take the Nurse Aide exam, you have taken the first step toward a great future! Of course, there is no point in taking this important examination unless you intend to do your very best in order to earn the highest grade you possibly can. That means getting yourself organized and discovering the best approaches, methods and strategies to master the material. Yes, that will require real effort and dedication on your part but if you are willing to focus your energy and devote the study time necessary, before you know it you will be opening that letter of acceptance for the job of your dreams.

We know that taking on a new endeavour can be a little scary, and it is easy to feel unsure of where to begin. That's where we come in. This study guide is designed to help you improve your test-taking skills, show you a few tricks of the trade and increase both your competency and confidence.

The Nurse Aide Exam

While we seek to make our guide as comprehensive as possible, it is important to note that like all exams, the Nurse Aide Exam might be adjusted at some future point. New material might be added, or content that is no longer relevant or applicable might be removed. It is always a good idea to give the materials you receive when you register to take the exam a careful review.

Practice Test 1

The practice test questions present questions that are representative of the type of question you should expect to find on a Nurse Aide exam. However, they are not intended to match exactly what is on the any Nurse Aide exam.

For the best results, take this Practice Test as if it were the real exam. Set aside time when you will not be disturbed, and a location that is quiet and free of distractions. Read the instructions carefully, read each question carefully, and answer to the best of your ability.

Use the bubble answer sheets provided. When you have completed the Practice Test, check your answer against the Answer Key and read the explanation provided.

Remember – the purpose of a practice test is to learn! After completing the first practice test, mark your answers, then go back and review the explanations to see where you went wrong.

Answer Sheet – Practice Test I

1. Ⓐ Ⓑ Ⓒ Ⓓ
2. Ⓐ Ⓑ Ⓒ Ⓓ
3. Ⓐ Ⓑ Ⓒ Ⓓ
4. Ⓐ Ⓑ Ⓒ Ⓓ
5. Ⓐ Ⓑ Ⓒ Ⓓ
6. Ⓐ Ⓑ Ⓒ Ⓓ
7. Ⓐ Ⓑ Ⓒ Ⓓ
8. Ⓐ Ⓑ Ⓒ Ⓓ
9. Ⓐ Ⓑ Ⓒ Ⓓ
10. Ⓐ Ⓑ Ⓒ Ⓓ
11. Ⓐ Ⓑ Ⓒ Ⓓ
12. Ⓐ Ⓑ Ⓒ Ⓓ
13. Ⓐ Ⓑ Ⓒ Ⓓ
14. Ⓐ Ⓑ Ⓒ Ⓓ
15. Ⓐ Ⓑ Ⓒ Ⓓ
16. Ⓐ Ⓑ Ⓒ Ⓓ
17. Ⓐ Ⓑ Ⓒ Ⓓ

18. Ⓐ Ⓑ Ⓒ Ⓓ
19. Ⓐ Ⓑ Ⓒ Ⓓ
20. Ⓐ Ⓑ Ⓒ Ⓓ
21. Ⓐ Ⓑ Ⓒ Ⓓ
22. Ⓐ Ⓑ Ⓒ Ⓓ
23. Ⓐ Ⓑ Ⓒ Ⓓ
24. Ⓐ Ⓑ Ⓒ Ⓓ
25. Ⓐ Ⓑ Ⓒ Ⓓ
26. Ⓐ Ⓑ Ⓒ Ⓓ
27. Ⓐ Ⓑ Ⓒ Ⓓ
28. Ⓐ Ⓑ Ⓒ Ⓓ
29. Ⓐ Ⓑ Ⓒ Ⓓ
30. Ⓐ Ⓑ Ⓒ Ⓓ
31. Ⓐ Ⓑ Ⓒ Ⓓ
32. Ⓐ Ⓑ Ⓒ Ⓓ
33. Ⓐ Ⓑ Ⓒ Ⓓ
34. Ⓐ Ⓑ Ⓒ Ⓓ

35. Ⓐ Ⓑ Ⓒ Ⓓ
36. Ⓐ Ⓑ Ⓒ Ⓓ
37. Ⓐ Ⓑ Ⓒ Ⓓ
38. Ⓐ Ⓑ Ⓒ Ⓓ
39. Ⓐ Ⓑ Ⓒ Ⓓ
40. Ⓐ Ⓑ Ⓒ Ⓓ
41. Ⓐ Ⓑ Ⓒ Ⓓ
42. Ⓐ Ⓑ Ⓒ Ⓓ
43. Ⓐ Ⓑ Ⓒ Ⓓ
44. Ⓐ Ⓑ Ⓒ Ⓓ
45. Ⓐ Ⓑ Ⓒ Ⓓ
46. Ⓐ Ⓑ Ⓒ Ⓓ
47. Ⓐ Ⓑ Ⓒ Ⓓ
48. Ⓐ Ⓑ Ⓒ Ⓓ
49. Ⓐ Ⓑ Ⓒ Ⓓ
50. Ⓐ Ⓑ Ⓒ Ⓓ

Case 1

Your supervisor has assigned you a patient, John, a 78-year-old man with Dementia. He fell out of his bed and sprained his wrist. He is diabetic and suffers from left-sided weakness due to a stroke. He requires total care and assistance with everything he does. He has dentures. He can no longer walk alone, feed himself, bathe or dress himself, and he is incontinent of urine and stool. His vital signs are to be monitored q 4 hrs.

1. You are preparing to shave John. You need to assemble your supplies. What is the first action you should take?

    a. Place a warm damp towel around his face to soften his beard and relax him

    b. Check the chart to see if you should shave him and if so what type of razor you can safely use.

    c. Gather your towels, razor and shaving cream and proceed to John's room

    d. Make certain John has the privacy required to perform ADL's

2. You have checked the chart and it is safe to shave John using a standard razor. You should

    a. Draw the razor in the direction of hair growth

    b. Draw the razor opposite the direction of hair growth

    c. Pull the skin taut

    d. Both a and d

3. In performing John's daily care, you note that his toenails need to be trimmed. You should do which of the following?

    a. Gather your supplies and carefully trim his nails after cleaning his feet.

    b. Ignore it

    c. Note it in your documentation so that a doctor can cut his nails

    d. Plan to trim his nails while you are bathing him

4. When should you clean John's dentures?

    a. Before performing mouth care or cleaning

    b. After performing mouth care or cleaning

    c. Every 2 hours

    d. Before and after each meal

5. Oral care of any type should be performed

    a. At least twice per day

    b. After each meal

    c. Before and after each meal

    d. After each meal, in the morning and each night before the patient goes to sleep

6. In order to make John's bed, which of the following will you need?

    a. Gloves

    b. Clean linens, gloves, and a bag for dirty linens

    c. Clean linens and a bag for dirty linens

    d. Clean linens

7. When removing your contaminated gloves after making John's bed, you would

a. Grasp the fingers of one glove using the other gloved hand and remove it

b. Grasp the cuff of one gloved had using the other gloved hand and remove it

c. Grasp the palm of one gloved hand using the other gloved hand and remove the glove leaving it in your remaining gloved hand. Then you would place your un-gloved fingers beneath the cuff of the remaining dirty glove, removing it by turning it inside out keeping the glove you have already removed inside the palm of the glove you are removing

d. Grasp the fingers of each glove and remove them by gently tugging at the ends and dispose of them in the appropriate receptacle

8. John has gone down to radiology for a chest x-ray. You decide to take advantage of the time to make his bed. The first thing you would do is

a. Strip the bed of dirty linens

b. Clear the room of visitors

c. Roll the dirty linens into a ball, carry them held away from your body and deposit them in the dirty linen bag

d. Maneuver the bed into its 'flat' position

9. The second thing you should do in preparing to make John's bed is to

a. Raise the bed to a comfortable working height

b. Remove the dirty linens

c. Gather your clean linens and other supplies

d. None of the above

10. When removing the dirty linens from John's bed you would do which of the following?

    a. You should just pull them off and carry them to the dirty linen bag and place them there

    b. Loosen them and roll each end toward the center and carry them to the dirty linen bag

    c. Remove each item individually and inspect it for blood and then take it to the dirty laundry bag

    d. It doesn't matter how you remove the linens as long as they are placed in the appropriate receptacle

11. After removing the dirty linens, you notice that John's mattress is soiled. You should

    a. Call and have the mattress replaced

    b. Document your findings

    c. Wipe the mattress down

    d. Make the bed and have it ready for John

12. When preparing to make John's bed, you notice that his glasses are on the bed. You should (Choose the MOST correct answer)

    a. Remove them while making the bed and place them on the bedside table

    b. Document your findings

    c. Put them in your pocket so that they will not get broken

    d. All of the above

13. The following day you are once again assigned to be John's caregiver. You are preparing to make his bed, but he cannot get up today. You must make the bed with him in it. It is best, when making an occupied bed if

    a. You can obtain assistance from a co-worker

    b. You get assistance from a family member

    c. Raise John's head to a 30 degree angle

    d. Document that you need to make the bed while John is in it

14. **John should be bathed**

    a. Daily
    b. Twice daily
    c. Only as needed
    d. None of the above

15. **In order to bathe John, you will need**

    a. Towels, three sheets, bath cloths, soap, warm water and a basin

    b. Towels, warm water, a basin, and soap

    c. Towels, wash cloths, a basin, soap and warm water

    d. Towels, a warm blanket, wash cloths, a basin, soap and warm water

16. You are going to bathe John. The MOST appropriate thing you should do is

    a. Provide for privacy

    b. Gather your supplies after making certain there is no one in the room but John

    c. Gather your supplies and then provide for John's privacy

    d. Bathe John as long as only family members are present

17. Bath water should be

    a. Changed if it cools

    b. Hot

    c. Soapy

    d. Changed between bathing of each body quadrant

18. You have prepared to bathe John. You are now washing his arms. You should

    a. Use slow circular strokes.

    b. Wash the arm proximal to distal

    c. Wash the arm distal to proximal

    d. Use short strokes away from the heart

19. The taking of John's vital signs includes

    a. Temperature, blood pressure, respirations. and pulse

    b. blood pressure, respirations, pulse and ROM

    c. temperature, I&O, respirations, pulse and blood pressure

    d. All of the above

20. When taking John's blood pressure, you should make certain that

    a. The cuff is the correct size
    b. John is lying on his left side
    c. The cuff is positioned dependent to his elbow
    d. The cuff is pumped to at least 20 mm above his baseline b/p

21. You will get the most accurate temperature

    a. Under the arm
    b. Rectally
    c. At the groin
    d. In the ear

22. When counting the pulse rate, what points should you use?

    a. The carotid artery
    b. The radial artery
    c. The apical area of the heart via the chest using a stethoscope
    d. All of the above

23. While assessing John's temperature, you note that it is 101.2 degrees. What is your FIRST action?

    a. Notify your supervisor
    b. Call the doctor
    c. Wait the appropriate amount of time and take the temperature again
    d. Have a co-worker check your work.

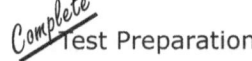

24. In order that John may be placed in the sitting position in bed, you should first

    a. Check with the charge nurse to make sure the doctor allows that position
    b. Ask someone to assist you in re-positioning him
    c. Clear the patient's room
    d. Take the patient's vital signs

25. You have gotten a co-worker to assist you in repositioning John to a sitting position in bed. Your next action should be to

    a. Lower the bed to a comfortable working height for both you and your assistant
    b. Grasp the draw sheet and count to 3, then lift/pull in the direction of the head of the bed
    c. Explain to John what you are going to do
    d. None of the above

26. You have gotten a co-worker to assist you in re-positioning John and you have explained to him what you are going to do. What is your next action?

    a. Lower the bed to a comfortable working height
    b. Reiterate to John what you will be doing
    c. Assess John's ability to assist you
    d. Grasp the draw sheet, count to 3, then lift/pull toward the top of the bed

27. John is preparing get up out of bed into a wheelchair for the first time after his admission. It is important to encourage him to sit on the side of the bed and dangle his feet for a while to ensure that

    a. Drops his blood pressure.
    b. Has enough will to get up out of bed
    c. Gets dizzy.
    d. He can tolerate the movement.

28. Should you decide to transport John by wheelchair, It is important to remember that you should push him from behind in all of the following scenarios except

    a. entering the elevator
    b. re-entering his room
    c. when you go into the cafeteria
    d. when you are going down the hall

29. When preparing to transfer John from his bed to the wheelchair you should

    a. position the chair at a 45 degree angle at his bedside
    b. position the chair at a 30 degree angle at his bedside and lock the wheels
    c. position the chair to a 45 degree angle at his bedside and lock the wheels
    d. position the chair at a 30 degree angle at his bedside

30. When transferring John to the wheelchair you should make certain that

    a. The wheelchair is sturdy
    b. You have the chair positioned at a 43 degree angle to the bed
    c. Most of the wheels are locked
    d. The bed is in its lowest position

31. When lifting, transferring or moving patients to a chair, the MOST important consideration is

   a.   Comfort
   b.   Documentation
   c.   Protocol
   d.   Safety

Case 2

Paul, a 45-year-old construction worker has been admitted to the hospital for surgery. The doctor has determined that he requires an ostomy. He has been assigned to you for care.

32. When providing ostomy care, you should

   a.   Clean the area around the stoma or ostomy site thoroughly with warm soap and water
   b.   Avoid the ostomy area and clean all surrounding areas thoroughly
   c.   Obtain assistance in cleaning the ostomy area
   d.   Avoid the use of soap on the ostomy area

33. An ostomy site is

   a.   An opening allowing for the exit of urine from the body
   b.   An opening allowing for the exit of stool from the body
   c.   An operative site which has been closed recently requiring frequent dressing changes
   d.   Both a and b

Case 3

Joyce is a 57 year old patient who has been assigned to you. She had surgery yesterday.

34. Joyce begins talking about the death of her sister to you. You should

    a. Listen
    b. Leave the room
    c. Tell her about the death of your brother
    d. Advise her to talk to her doctor

35. It is appropriate for you to share the information regarding a Joyce's status with

    a. Any one the nurse aide sees fit
    b. The client's family members
    c. The client's roommate
    d. The staff on the next shift

36. Joyce has developed redness and skin breakdown under her right wrist restraint. If you do not report this occurrence and report it, you are guilty of

    a. Negligence
    b. Slander
    c. Assault
    d. Threatening a patient

37. Upon entering Joyce's room, you note that a laboratory technician is attempting to perform to draw blood. He is holding Joyce's arm down forcibly while she is trying to pull away and is calling for help. The tech is guilty of

    a. Slander
    b. Assault
    c. Nothing
    d. None of the above

38. Joyce requires the use of the bedpan. You should

   a. Turn her on her side with knees flexed
   b. Ask him to lift her hips and place the bedpan beneath his buttocks
   c. Raise her head to a 30 degree angle
   d. None of the above

39. After Joyce has used the bedpan, you should

   a. Empty and rinse the bedpan and store it appropriately
   b. Clean her skin with disposable wipes and dry it
   c. Both a and b
   d. None of the above

40. The doctor has ordered an enema for Joyce. Which of the following do you need to assemble?

   a. Bedpan, incontinence pads, gloves, a pre-prepared enema solution or hospital approved enema equipment, and lubricating solution
   b. Warm water, pads, a bedpan, gloves and an apron
   c. The enema solution, lubricating jell, and incontinence pads
   d. Just the enema solution

41. You should position Joyce

   a. Supine
   b. Lying on her right side
   c. Lying on her left side
   d. Lying on her stomach

42. The Kubler-Ross stages of grief include

   a. Denial, anger and bargaining
   b. Acceptance, bargaining and denial
   c. Depression, anger, acceptance, crying and denial
   d. Denial, anger, bargaining, depression and acceptance

43. Which of the following behavior is not a sign or a symptom of anxiety?

   a. Frequent hand movement
   b. Somatization
   c. The client asks a question
   d. The client is acting out

44. Joyce is angry because of the addition of restraints. What skill would you use to deal with her angry outbursts?

   a. Listening
   b. Advising
   c. Restating
   d. None of the above

45. While dealing with Joyce's bouts of anger, she becomes belligerent and her language toward you is abusive. The proper manner in which to deal with her behavior is

   a. To remain calm
   b. Walk out of the room and tell your co-worker what has occurred so that you can't be sued
   c. Advise Joyce that her behavior is not acceptable
   d. Both a and c

46. A person who is _____ may indicate the desire to place an unconscious barrier between themselves and others.

   a. Avoiding eye contact
   b. Yawning widely
   c. Making wild gestures
   d. Crossing their arms across their chest

47. When communicating with another person, _____ is/are used to emphasize an important point, _____ can indicate either great interest or boredom, and _____ can express encouragement or empathy.

a. When communicating with another person, gestures are used to emphasize an important point, posture can indicate either great interest or boredom, and touch can express encouragement or empathy.

b. When communicating with another person, touch is used to emphasize an important point, posture can indicate either great interest or boredom, and gestures can express encouragement or empathy.

c. When communicating with another person, posture is used to emphasize an important point, gestures can indicate either great interest or boredom, and touch can express encouragement or empathy.

d. When communicating with another person, gestures are used to emphasize an important point, touch can indicate either great interest or boredom, and posture can express encouragement or empathy.

48. Which, if any, of the following statements about eye contact are false?

    a.   Consistent eye contact can indicate a positive reaction to a speaker.

    b.   Consistent eye contact can indicate a lack of trust in the speaker.

    c.   The use of eye contact may be dependent on the culture of the listener.

    d.   None of these statements are false.

49. _____ is a technique used to put people at ease.

    a. Speaking softly
    b. Making eye contact
    c. Mirroring body language
    d. Leaning forward

50. Which, if any, of these statements about body language are false?

    a. Everyone uses some form of body language to communicate.
    b. Interpretations of body language are universal to all cultures.
    c. The study of body language is called kinetic interpretation.
    d. Indications of emotion such as smiling when happy are universal.

51. _____ can signal a lack of interest or an unfriendly attitude and can make therapeutic communication difficult to achieve.

    a. Eye contact
    b. Questioning
    c. Empathy
    d. Nonverbal communication

52. If a patient asks a question that is beyond the scope of your practice, the best response would be to:

    a. Make your best guess based on what you know.
    b. Tell the patient that you will find them the correct answer.
    c. Change the subject.
    d. Give them a book on the subject.

53. What is the recommended method of turning off a hand faucet after washing your hands?

   a. After applying lotion
   a. With a paper or cloth towel
   b. After putting on surgical gloves
   c. None of the Above

54. The most important standard precaution is

   a. Treat all bodily fluids as contaminated
   b. Wear gloves as much as possible
   c. Only wear gloves when you think a patient is contaminated
   d. Always label specimens immediately

55. What federal agency develops and monitors standards for workplace health and safety?

   a. FDA
   b. ADA
   c. OSHA
   d. None of the Above

56. Influenza is caused by

   a. A fungus
   b. Bacteria
   c. A virus
   d. Protozoa

57. A (n) _____ _____ is a legal document filed in advance by a patient which details their wishes in the event that they are incapacitated.

   a. Last will and testament
   b. Beneficiary list
   c. Advance directive
   d. Funeral plan

58. Which if any of the following statements about living wills is true?

a. They state the type of care a patient does or does not want to receive at the end of their life.
b. They are documents in which the patient chooses a surrogate who can make healthcare decisions in the event that they are incapacitated.
c. They demand that no extraordinary measures such as CPR, are used in an effort to revive the patient.
d. All of the above.

59. What are the two types of advance directives?

a. A durable power of attorney and a DNR order
b. A funeral plan and a living will
c. A life insurance policy and a durable power of attorney
d. A living will and a durable power of attorney

60. Maintaining _____ requires that information about a patient's current medical status, treatments and discussion of further treatment is only used for its intended purpose.

a. Confidentiality
b. Privacy
c. Discretion
d. Autonomy

Quick Reference Answer Key

1. A	31. D
2. D	32. A
3. C	33. D
4. A	34. A
5. D	35. D
6. B	36. A
7. C	37. B
8. D	38. A
9. A	39. C
10. B	40. A
11. C	41. C
12. A	42. D
13. A	43. C
14. A	44. A
15. D	45. C
16. C	46. D
17. A	47. A
18. C	48. D
19. A	49. C
20. A	50. C
21. B	51. D
22. D	52. B
23. C	53. B
24. B	54. A
25. C	55. C
26. C	56. C
27. D	57. C
28. A	58. D
29. C	59. D
30. D	60. A

Answer Key with Explanations

1. A
You should always make certain a patient can be shaved and what type of razor is appropriate. If a patient is septic, it may be dangerous for the patient if you shave him at all. Shaving risks a cut that could cause issues with his already compromised immune system.

2. D
You should always shave in the direction of hair growth which changes depending on where you are shaving. Pulling the shin taut allows shaving with minimal risk of cutting.

3. C
The only person who can trim a diabetics nails is a doctor due to potential for infection.

4. A
The appropriate sequence when administering mouth care to a person with dentures is to clean the dentures first. Then you should perform oral care or cleaning. The dentures are then clean and ready for the patient as soon as you have completed oral care.

5. D
Oral care is an essential part of appropriate nursing care. You should give oral care frequently during the day in order to maintain good oral health.

6. B
You always need gloves when removing dirty linens or performing other tasks which could bring your skin into contact with pathogens or body fluids. Clean linens and a bag for dirty laundry are essential.

7. C
The gloves are removed in such a manner that your skin does not come into contact with contaminated areas of the

gloves and they are turned so that one is contained within the other and appropriately disposed of.

8. D
Unoccupied beds are always made up while in the flat position. Doing so ensures a nice smooth bed which will not irritate the skin. Additionally, it is easier to work with a bed in the flat position than with the head or foot raised.

9. A
You should always observe good body mechanics when working. Raising the bed to a comfortable working height ensures less back strain.

10. B
Dirty linens are always rolled toward the center, keeping any contaminants contained, and placed in the dirty linen bag.

11. C
Part of your duties when making a bed, whether occupied or unoccupied is to make certain that everything, including the mattress, is clean.

12. A
The patient's belongings should always be left in the room where they can easily be located by the patient.

13. A
It is safer for John and will promote more efficient care if you have assistance. Shifting John for changing linens can be difficult physically for one person if the patient is unable to assist you.

14. A
A patient should be bathed daily and then cleaned as needed between each bath.

15. D
You will need clean towels, soap and water and a basin of course. You will also need a blanket to cover John for privacy and dignity and to provide warmth while you bathe him.

16. C
John is entitled to privacy while receiving a bath. Family members are no exception. If you wait until after you provide for privacy to gather your equipment, it may be necessary to empty the room again of visitors.

17. A
Water should be maintained at a comfortable temperature for bathing. It should always be changed and replaced with warm water if it cools.

18. C
Hands and arms are always washed distal to proximal. You should always wash from cleanest to dirtiest. The armpit is considered dirty. In addition, you should always wash the patient using strokes that lead toward the heart. This increases venous return.

19. A
The four components of the vital sign assessment are temperature, blood pressure, pulse, and respirations.

20. A
If the cuff is not the proper width for your patient, you will get a false reading on your blood pressure check.

21. B
The rectal temperature is taken within the body cavity and therefore yields a temperature reading closest to actual body temperature.

22. D
The pulse can accurately be counted using any of these areas, although for most initial assessments the radial pulse is used.

23. C
Always double-check your vital signs to make certain there is a valid problem.

24. B
When repositioning a patient, it is always in the best interest of the patient and the nurse to obtain assistance. This

allows for safety for both.

25. C
Never attempt to perform an action for the patient without first explaining what you are going to do and how you will be going about it.

26. C
The MOST appropriate answer is c. You should always allow the patient to do whatever they can to assist in their own care. Never exclude them!

27. D
Many things occur within the body when position is changed; blood pressure may rise or fall. The patient is most likely already weakened from having been bed bound. While the patient is sitting bedside, you can evaluate his ability to move safely.

28. A
A wheelchair bound patient is always turned facing outward and backed into an elevator. This prevents disorientation and dizziness on the part of the patient as well as promoting the use of good body mechanics for the nurse.

29. C
A 45-degree angle allows space to assist your patient in the transfer but not so much that you can't stabilize him is he slips. A 30-degree angle would be too wide to allow for control over a fall. Wheelchair wheels are ALWAYS locked.

30. D
The bed must be in the lowest position possible for both the safety of the patient as well as the nurse. Try to get the area we are transferring the patient from as close as possible. This will enable us to 'pivot' with John rather than manually carry him to his wheelchair.

31. D
The safety of both patient and nurse is foremost in the transferring of patients.

32. A
The skin surrounding the ostomy site must be kept clean and dry. Enzymes from exudate can erode the skin if proper care is not implemented.

33. D
An ostomy is used to allow for the exit of feces and urine when a patient's body can no longer perform this function normally.

34. A
You need to listen when your patient begins to talk about loss. It is part of your therapeutic intervention as a professional.

35. D
Staff members involved with your patient's care are the only ones you can share information. Giving report to the next shift is appropriate.

36. A
If you do not address the change in status of a patient, but rather ignore it, you are guilty of professional negligence and can be held accountable.

37. B
Assault is the unauthorized or forcible touching of another person.

38. A
When preparing to place a patient on the bedpan, you should have him/her positioned on one side with knees flexed, place the bedpan beneath the buttocks and have them roll over onto the bedpan using their flexed knees to lift their hips and position themselves comfortably on the bedpan.

39. C
Skin care is always provided after bedpan use to prevent tissue breakdown. You must always empty and rinse the bedpan and store it appropriately after use.

40. A
You would need all of this equipment in order to perform the enema, protect yourself and the patient's linens and to lubricate the anal opening for ease of entry.

41. C
The patient is positioned on the left side in order to facilitate entry of the enema fluid into the colon. The colon is situated within the abdomen such that the flow of the enema fluid from this position would enter the rectum flowing naturally into the descending colon and on across the transverse colon to the ascending colon.

42. D
The five phases of this grief model include denial, anger, bargaining, depression and acceptance.

43. C
If the client is asking questions, they are coping with feelings. All of the other answers are symptoms of an anxious patient.

44. A
In order to address the reason for her anger, you must listen to why she is angry.

45. C
It is appropriate to advise a patient that abusive behavior is unacceptable. Above all, you MUST remain calm and professional.

46. D
A person who is **crossing their arms across their chest** may indicate the desire to place an unconscious barrier between themselves and others.

47. A
When communicating with another person, gestures are used to emphasize an important point, posture can indicate either great interest or boredom, and touch can express encouragement or empathy.

48. D
None of these statements are false.
Consistent eye contact can indicate a positive reaction to a speaker.

Consistent eye contact can indicate a lack of trust in the speaker.

The use of eye contact may be dependent on the culture of the listener.

49. C
The idea of mirroring body language to put people at ease is commonly used in interviews. Mirroring the body language indicates that they are understood.

50. C
The study of body language is called kinetic interpretation is false.

51. D
Nonverbal communication can signal a lack of interest or an unfriendly attitude, and can make therapeutic communication difficult to achieve.

52. B
If a patient asks a question and you do not know the answer, the best response is the response that is the most helpful. I.e. that you will assist them in finding the answer. Saying that you don't know or similar responses are not helpful to the patient.

53. B
Turning off the tap with a paper towel prevents contamination from the tap.

54. A
The most important standard precaution is **to treat all bodily fluids as contaminated.**

55. C
The United States Occupational Safety and Health Administration (OSHA) is an agency of the United States Department of Labor. Its mission is to prevent work-related in-

juries, illnesses, and occupational fatality by issuing and enforcing standards for workplace safety and health.

56. C
Influenza, commonly referred to as the flu, is an infectious disease caused by RNA viruses of the family Orthomyxoviridae (the influenza viruses), that affects birds and mammals. The most common symptoms of the disease are chills, fever, sore throat, muscle pains, severe headache, coughing, weakness/fatigue and general discomfort. Although it is often confused with other influenza-like illnesses, especially the common cold, influenza is a more severe disease than the common cold and is caused by a different type of virus.[1]

57. C
An **advance directive** is a legal document filed in advance by a patient which details their wishes in the event that they are incapacitated.

An advance health care directive, also known as living will, personal directive, advance directive, or advance decision, are instructions given by individuals specifying what actions should be taken for their health in the event that they are no longer able to make decisions due to illness or incapacity, and appoints a person to make such decisions on their behalf. A living will is one form of advance directive, leaving instructions for treatment. Another form authorizes a specific type of power of attorney or health care proxy, where someone is appointed by the individual to make decisions on their behalf when they are incapacitated. People may also have a combination of both. It is often encouraged that people complete both documents to provide the most comprehensive guidance regarding their care. One example of a combination document is the Five Wishes advance directive in the United States.[2]

58. D
The following are true about living wills:

They are documents in which the patient chooses a surrogate who can make healthcare decisions in the event that they are incapacitated.

They demand that no extraordinary measures such as CPR, are used in an effort to revive the patient.

59. D
Two types of advance directives are **a living will and a durable power of attorney.**

An advance health care directive, also known as living will, personal directive, advance directive, or advance decision, are instructions given by individuals specifying what actions should be taken for their health in the event that they are no longer able to make decisions due to illness or incapacity, and appoints a person to make such decisions on their behalf. A living will is one form of advance directive, leaving instructions for treatment. Another form authorizes a specific type of power of attorney or health care proxy, where the individual appoints someone to make decisions on their behalf when they are incapacitated. People may also have a combination of both. It is often encouraged that people complete both documents to provide the most comprehensive guidance regarding their care. One example of a combination document is the Five Wishes advance directive in the United States.[2]

60. A
Maintaining confidentiality requires that information about a patient's current medical status, treatments and discussion of further treatment is only used for its intended purpose.

Practice Test 2

The practice test presents questions representative of questions you can expect to find on a Nurse Aide exam. However, they are not intended to match exactly what is on any particular exam.

For the best results, take this Practice Test as if it were the real exam. Set aside time when you will not be disturbed, and a location that is quiet and free of distractions. Read the instructions carefully, read each question carefully, and answer to the best of your ability.

Use the bubble answer sheets provided. When you have completed the Practice Test, check your answer against the Answer Key and read the explanation provided.

Answer Sheet – Practice Test II

1. A B C D
2. A B C D
3. A B C D
4. A B C D
5. A B C D
6. A B C D
7. A B C D
8. A B C D
9. A B C D
10. A B C D
11. A B C D
12. A B C D
13. A B C D
14. A B C D
15. A B C D
16. A B C D
17. A B C D
18. A B C D
19. A B C D
20. A B C D
21. A B C D
22. A B C D
23. A B C D
24. A B C D
25. A B C D
26. A B C D
27. A B C D
28. A B C D
29. A B C D
30. A B C D
31. A B C D
32. A B C D
33. A B C D
34. A B C D
35. A B C D
36. A B C D
37. A B C D
38. A B C D
39. A B C D
40. A B C D
41. A B C D
42. A B C D
43. A B C D
44. A B C D
45. A B C D
46. A B C D
47. A B C D
48. A B C D
49. A B C D
50. A B C D

1. When performing a patient's oral care, you should first

   a.   Place his head at a 45 degree angle

   b.   Place his head flat and have him turn his head to one side

   c.   Have him swish his mouth with mouthwash

   d.   Clean the inside of his mouth using gentle circular motions

2. Patient's oral care should include

   a.   Denture care

   b.   Gentle cleaning of the oral mucosa and lips

   c.   Cleaning of the tongue

   d.   All of the above

3. Your co-worker tells you that the doctor has ordered cold packs for a patient's sprained wrist. You are aware that

   a.   You should assess their skin before applying the pack and document your findings

   b.   The cold pack should be applied for no longer than twenty minutes per interval

   c.   You should read the order thoroughly prior to administering the cold pack.

   d.   All of the above

4. After applying the cold pack, you should reassess the patient's skin

   a.   Every 5 minutes

   b.   Every 10 minutes

   c.   As often as you can

   d.   Only after the 20 minute treatment has been completed

5. After application of the cold pack you should

   a.   Document that the order was carried out, the skin condition before and after application and the duration of the treatment

   b.   Document that the order was carried out and sign the chart

   c.   Remove the cold pack and properly dispose of it and tell your co-worker that you have completed the treatment

   d.   All of the above

6. Your co-worker has rolled John onto his right side. The top sheet has been removed. In order to remove the bottom layers and replace them you would

   a.   Roll the dirty linen from the edge of the bed inward toward John.

   b.   Roll the dirty linen from the top toward John's waist making certain that the dirty side is rolled toward the center then roll the remaining linen from John's feet toward the center taking the same care to keep the dirty side toward the center

   c.   Pull the dirty linen out from under John's body and place it in the dirty linen bag

   d.   Place the clean linen on top of the soiled linen and then remove the dirty linen appropriately placing in the dirty linen container

7. Should you determine that John can assist you safely, when preparing to change John's linens you would

   a.   Lower the bedrail on the side opposite you leaving the other rail raised while working

   b.   Lower the bedrail closest to you leaving the other rail raised while working

   c.   Lower both bedrails while working

   d.   Lower the bed to its lowest position prior to beginning

8. It is necessary to keep John covered while you are making his bed

   a. Only if there are others in the room
   b. At all times
   c. If the room is cool
   d. Until you get the draw sheet in place

9. When making John's bed, you have replaced the bottom linens on your side. Your coworker is preparing to complete the change of linens. You assist John in rolling over. Your co-worker would then

   a. Grasp the roll of clean linens and unroll them from center toward the side of the bed making certain they were smooth and wrinkle free
   b. Grasp the linens and pull hard so that the linens will be wrinkle free
   c. Raise the bed rail
   d. Place clean linens under John making certain they were wrinkle free.

10. After you have completed making John's bed, you should wash your hands. The proper manner in which you would do this is

   a. Wash your hands using plenty of warm water and soap, thoroughly rinse and dry
   b. Wash your hands, including cleaning your nails, using plenty of warm soap and water, rinse and dry
   c. Wash your hands, including nails, using warm water and soap, rinse and dry
   d. Wash your hands and clean your nails using warm water and soap, rinse and dry using your towel to turn off the water

11. You should wash your hands

  a. 4 times daily
  b. Before and after patient contact
  c. When they become soiled
  d. Both b and c

12. You have placed John in a semi-sitting position. The head of his bed is at 45 degrees. This position is called

  a. Recumbent
  b. Flexed
  c. Sim's
  d. Fowler's

13. John is lying on his side with his thigh flexed. The doctor is preparing to perform a rectal examination. This position is appropriately named

  a. Fowler's
  b. Freud's
  c. Sim's
  d. Sam's

14. When bathing John, you should

  a. ALWAYS use soap, clean towels and warm water
  b. Use firms strokes in the direction of the heart
  c. Rub briskly with your cloth in order to stimulate circulation
  d. Wait until later in your day because it will take a long time to bathe him

15. When dressing John you should always

   a.   Let him do what he can on his own and assist with what he can't do
   b.   Do everything for him
   c.   Insist that he dress himself because it is therapeutic for him to be independent
   d.   Get someone to assist you

16. You have completed John's bath and are preparing to dress him. You have provided a clean shirt. In order to put his shirt on, which arm should you put into the sleeve first?

   a.   Both
   b.   Left
   c.   Right
   d.   Let John choose

17. A back massage is

   a.   Not a part of the bathing duties
   b.   The time when skin assessment can be made
   c.   Included in bathing
   d.   Both b and c

18. Bathing is performed in order to

   a.   Remove bacteria from the skin surface
   b.   Promote relaxation
   c.   Improve circulation
   d.   All of the above

19. You are going to transfer John from his bed to a chair. You have placed the chair at the appropriate angle and the bed is in lowest potion. Which of the following is the BEST way to complete the transfer?

   a. Using your back and arms, pull John upright and pivot toward the chair and gently settle him into the chair
   b. Wrapping your arms around John's torso and with knees slightly bent; use your legs to turn with the patient. Ask the patient, if he is capable, to grasp the arm of the chair. If now, slowly back toward the chair until you feel with your own leg that it is there. Slowly lower John into the chair.
   c. Using only your arms and legs, lift the patient into your arms and settle him safely into his chair.
   d. Obtain assistance from a co-worker. Each of you take one side of the patient and gently lift, using proper body mechanics, and transfer him to his chair.

20. What is the rationale for getting a patient out of bed?

   a. in order to maintain muscle tone
   b. To improve muscle tone
   c. To allow for adequate pulmonary function
   d. All of the above

21. Which of the following is NOT a stage of assisting a patient in getting out of bed safely?

   a. Assist the patient to stand
   b. Allow John to dangle his feet over the side of the bed
   c. Assist John in moving to the chair
   d. Asking a family member to explain to John what you are about to do

22. Which would you do first when assisting John out of bed?

    a. Assist him to a standing position

    b. Allow him to dangle his feet over the edge of the bed

    c. Move the chair out of his way

    d. Obtain the chair from across the room

23. John is being transferred to a chair. You and a co-worker are assisting him. Which part of your anatomy should be MOST involved in the transfer?

    a. Legs
    b. Back
    c. Arms and shoulders
    d. Both b and c

24. If John begins to become off balance or unstable during the transfer, you should

    a. Attempt to stabilize the patient by bracing him against you and guide the patient to the bedside or chair, if possible.

    b. If a fall begins to occur, guide him slowly toward the floor.

    c. Move back and allow the patient to slide to the floor and call for assistance

    d. Both a and b

25. If a fall occurs, as you gently glide your patient to the floor you should

    a. Protect his head
    b. Protect his IV
    c. Protect his drains
    d. Protect his extremities

26. After a John's fall, the first thing you should do is

a. Call for assistance in getting John off the floor and into bed or his chair
b. Just pick him up and complete the move
c. Assess for injuries and call for assistance
d. Talk to your assistant about what went wrong

27. After John's fall, what document must you fill out?

a. And incident report
b. The I & O sheet
c. Charting of the people who witnessed the fall
d. The vital sign flow sheet

28. While walking by a co-worker, you overhear her telling another worker that you have not addressed a patient's restraint care in your documentation. You are aware that this is untrue and that you have done all that you should do for your patient. Your co-worker's behavior is an example of

a. Slander
b. Assault
c. Defamation
d. Both a and d

29. After coming on duty later in the course of a patient's care, you note that her restraints have been tied to the bed frame. You are aware that this can cause injury to the patient and is inappropriate use of her restraints. This is an example of

a. Assault
b. Negligence
c. Appropriate action
d. Slander

30. You have just walked into a patient's room and you overhear a lab technician telling her to allow him to draw her blood or he will tighten her restraints. The lab tech is guilty of

   a. Slander
   b. Threatening a patient
   c. Acting in the patient's best interest
   d. Violation of Joyce's privacy

31. Restraints may be used

   a. To force her to obey doctor's orders no matter what
   b. Only at night
   c. In accordance with doctor's orders only
   d. None of the above

32. All of the following are inappropriate within the scope of the hospital setting EXCEPT

   a. Documentation
   b. Providing for patient privacy
   c. Talking about a co-worker
   d. Using gloves

33. A patient has become confused and her doctor has ordered wrist restraints. All of the following are true of restraints except

   a. They should allow as much freedom of movement as possible
   b. They should be removed periodically
   c. Their application should be documented
   d. They should be tied to the bed frame

34. The patient has attempted to get out of bed and has managed to slip despite her wrist restraints. The doctor orders the addition of ankle restraints. You know that

    a. The use of restraints on all four extremities is also termed 'four point restraints'
    b. Range of motion exercises should be performed regularly
    c. You should observe for skin breakdown
    d. All of the above

35. Prior to application of the patient's ankle restraints, she kicked the side rail bruising her knee and causing minor swelling. The doctor has ordered that a cold pack be applied to the area. You would know that

    a. The cold pack will help with swelling and pain as well as bruising
    b. You should leave the cold pack in place no longer than 20 minutes
    c. You should assess the skin prior to applying the cold pack
    d. All of the above

36. Before you apply the patient's cold pack, you assess her skin integrity, temperature and color. You note that the skin is extremely cold, blue-black in color in an area extending beyond the damaged originally damaged area, the tissue is extremely swollen and Joyce is complaining of intense pain. You should

    a. Not apply the cold pack until you have reported your findings to the charge nurse or doctor
    b. Go ahead and apply the cold pack
    c. Initiate a CODE BLUE
    d. Gently massage the area prior to applying the cold pack

37. While assessing John's temperature, you note that it is 101.2 degrees. What is your FIRST action?

   a. Notify your supervisor
   b. Call the doctor
   c. Wait the appropriate amount of time and take the temperature again
   d. Have a co-worker check your work.

38. You can count respirations while

   a. Taking John's b/p
   b. Counting John's pulse
   c. Taking his temperature
   d. None of the above

39. When assessing John's respirations you should

   a. Count the number of times his chest rises and falls in one minute
   b. Auscultate his chest
   c. Observe whether John is breathing easily or seems to be having difficulty
   d. All of the above

40. If John's 3 year old granddaughter was visiting and was watching you take her grandfather's vital signs and became curious about how you would take hers, you might explain to her that

   a. You would do it on the arm but with a smaller cuff
   b. You would do it on her thigh but with a smaller cuff
   c. You would do it on her ankle using a smaller cuff
   d. All of the above.

41. You came on duty at 7 A.M. It is now 1 P.M. Assuming everything is normal, how many times should you have assessed John's vital sign status?

   a. Twice
   b. Once
   c. PRN
   d. Not at all

42. After assessing John's vitals, the MOST proper way to document them would be

   a. Bp140/72, Pulse regular and bounding, Respirations 16 and shallow, temp. 99.0
   b. Temp 99.0 orally, BP 140/72, Pulse regular, Respirations 16
   c. Pulse regular and bounding, Temp. 99.0 orally, B/P140/72, Respirations 16 and shallow
   d. None of the above

43. When taking a rectal temperature you will need

   a. Gloves and lubricant
   b. An oral thermometer
   c. A rectal thermometer
   d. Both a and c

44. In reviewing the care that you have administered to Joyce today, you are aware that her anger may have been

   a. A stage of grief
   b. Caused by her dislike of you
   c. Caused by a hereditary disease
   d. Temporary insanity

45. In order to assist Joyce in accepting the loss of her family member you must

   a. Read everything on death and dying before approaching her
   b. Be willing to talk with her about death
   c. Not bring up her loss, no matter what
   d. Distract her with conversation about other things

46. James, a 19-year-old college student has been admitted to the hospital for sports injuries sustained during a hockey game. He has been assigned to you. When you enter his room to take him his breakfast tray, he comments on your appearance and tries to touch you. You should

   a. Tell him that his actions are inappropriate
   b. Ignore him
   c. Slap his hand
   d. Call for help

47. After telling James that his actions are inappropriate, he apologizes and you leave the room. You should

   a. Document the occurrence and your response
   b. Call the police
   c. Talk to your co-workers to obtain support
   d. Ignore the incident

48. Joyce's family has been in to visit her. They have told her that her sister was killed in an automobile accident. While performing her care, you note that she is silent and withdrawn. You would know that this she is experiencing which of the Kubler-Ross stages of grief?

   a. Acceptance
   b. Denial
   c. Bargaining
   d. Depression

49. _____ is restating something that a patient has said, usually in fewer words and with emphasis on the main points of their statement.

   a. Attending
   b. Paraphrasing
   c. Clarifying
   d. Perception checking

50. Facial expression, posture and tone of voice are elements of _____.

   a. Open-ended questions
   b. Nonverbal communication
   c. Orientation process
   d. Good manners

51. Which, if any, of the following statements about nonverbal communication are true?

   a. Nonverbal communications are less reliable that verbal communication
   b. Nonverbal communications remain the same, regardless of ethnicity or culture.
   c. Nonverbal communications always send a clear message.
   d. Nonverbal communications can emphasize or contradict verbal messages.

52. _____ provides encourages the patient to continue talking without indicating agreement or disagreement.

   a. Smiling
   b. Leaning forward
   c. Nodding
   d. Paraphrasing

53. Using phrases that address a person's feelings, such as "You must be worried about your headaches," demonstrates _____.

   a. Empathy
   b. Interest
   c. Acceptance
   d. Recognition

54. When dealing with elderly patients, always _____.

   a. Use their first names to establish intimacy.
   b. Direct your questions to their caregivers.
   c. Speak loudly and distinctly.
   d. Address them as Miss, Mrs., or Mr., followed by their last name.

55. When interviewing a patient with a hearing loss, remember to _____.

   a. Speak slowly and look directly at the patient.
   b. Ensure that the room is brightly lit.
   c. Write down your questions and have them write their answers.
   d. Both a) and b).

56. A/an _____ is a form that is filled out as soon as possible following an event such as an injury to a patient.

   a. Tort
   b. Occurrence statement
   c. Testimonial
   d. Incident report

57. Using neutral remarks such as, "I see" and "I hear what you're saying" indicate _____ to the patient.

    a. Empathy
    b. Recognition
    c. Understanding
    d. Avoidance

58. If a patient refuses to make eye contact, you may find that they are _____.

    a. From a culture that considers direct eye contact rude.
    b. Very tired.
    c. Lying about their symptoms.
    d. Disinterested in the conversation.

59. When communicating with non-English speaking patients, professionals should:

    a. Repeat sentences word-for-word if the patient does not understand.
    b. Use their children as interpreters.
    c. Raise the volume of their voices.
    d. Immediately employ the services of an interpreter.

60. Which, if any, of the following statements about geriatrics are false?

    a. Geriatrics is a branch of medicine in which the focus is health care for the aging population.
    b. Geriatrics differs from gerontology, which is the study of the aging process itself.
    c. A geriatrician's practice is limited to persons over the age of 65.
    d. None of the above.

Quick Reference Answer Key

1. A
2. D
3. D
4. B
5. A
6. A
7. B
8. B
9. A
10. D
11. D
12. D
13. C
14. B
15. A
16. B
17. D
18. D
19. B
20. D
21. D
22. B
23. A
24. A
25. A
26. C
27. A
28. D
29. B
30. B

31. C
32. C
33. D
34. D
35. D
36. A
37. C
38. C
39. D
40. D
41. A
42. B
43. D
44. A
45. B
46. A
47. A
48. D
49. B
50. B
51. D
52. C
53. A
54. D
55. A
56. D
57. C
58. A
59. A
60. C

Answer Key with Explanations

1. A
Always place the head at this angle to prevent choking.

2. D
Mouth care includes all areas of the mouth both inside and out.

3. D
You never take an order from another person. Always check the chart yourself and read the order. You should assess skin integrity at every opportunity, especially with diabetics. Cold packs are NEVER left in place longer than 20 minutes.

4. B
You should always reassess skin 10 minutes after the application of a cold pack.

5. A
You should always document after a procedure is carried out. Note everything that you can about the area of treatment both before treatment is performed and afterward.

6. A
Always roll dirty linen toward the center to contain contaminates.

7. B
Lowering the rail nearest you allows you to work and leaving the opposite rail raised provide for John's safety by preventing a fall from the bed.

8. B
You should always keep a clean sheet, blanket or bath blanket over the patient even when replacing top linens. This is done to provide for warmth and privacy.

9. A
The linens are already under John, the bedrail should already be down, and you do not pull hard on linens that

a patient is lying on as this could injure the patient.

10. D
You would use the paper towel utilized to dry your hands to turn off the water avoiding contamination of your clean hands.

11. D
Hand washing is a critical part of patient care and personal safety.

12. D
Fowler's positioning is considered to be an upright position of varying degrees.

13. C
Sim's position is a side lying position with the patient's thigh flexed. This position facilitates access to the rectum and vagina for examination.

14. B
You can't always use soap, especially with geriatric patients. You should ALWAYS use strokes that travel in the direction heading toward the heart as this increases venous return.

15. A
Allowing John to do what he can promotes independence and dignity in a difficult situation. Offer assistance when needed.

16. B
When a patient has weakness in an extremity, that extremity is always dressed first.

17. D
A gentle back massage is part of the bathing process and allows inspection of the skin on the back and buttocks as well as documentation and reporting of any adverse findings.

18. D
The removal of bacteria, relaxation and improved circulation are all benefits of bathing.

19. B
None of the other answers take into account the proper use of body mechanics except for answer d. Answer d is incorrect because this exercise involves a one on one move....not an assisted move.

20. D
It is critical, if proper functioning of body systems is to be secured, that movement be encouraged as soon as feasible. Extended time as a bed-bound patient impairs normal system functioning.

21. D
You should be the one explaining what is happening to John.

22. B
You must allow John to dangle his feet over the edge of the bed for a short time. This allows for settling of equilibrium, blood pressure changes to settle, and blood flow to extremities time to alter.

23. A
Carry the majority of the force of the move on your legs. This prevents damage to the nurses back, arms and shoulders. All play a role in the transfer, but carry the bulk of the weight on your legs.

24. A
Should a fall begin to occur, your first priority is to protect the patient. Stabilize him with your body by bracing him against you and if it is impossible to avoid a fall then your only alternative is to guide him, gently to the floor.

25. A
The correct answer is to protect John's head. IV's, drains and extremities are all important, but a head blow could be very serious, even lethal.

26. C
Of course, you will need assistance in getting him off the floor, but your first priority is in ascertaining whether

John has sustained injuries due to the fall. You should NOT move him further without both assistance and assessment.

27. A
Whenever an unexpected occurrence happens which involves a patient, or even a worker, you MUST fill out an incident report.

28. D
Your co-worker has spoken about you to others and the things said were untrue and could damage your reputation and endanger your license.

29. B
Properly trained medical personnel know that a hospital bed is created to move. Tying restraints to the bed will injure a patient at some point when the position of the bed is changed and must be avoided.

30. B
The tech has threatened Joyce with action he is not authorized to perform and which may cause her fear and anxiety in order to elicit her cooperation. This is inappropriate behavior.

31. C
Forcing a patient to do anything using restraints constitutes abuse and negligence. You must only use restraints in accordance with her doctor's orders.

32. C
Talking about a co-worker can constitute slander and defamation of character. At the least, it is unprofessional conduct and you should avoid.

33. D
A, b, and c are all true of the appropriate use of restraints. Tying the restraint off to the bed frame places the patient in jeopardy if the position of the bed is changed.

34. D
You always perform ROM exercises on restrained limbs

regularly and the potential for skin breakdown is increased with the addition of restraints. The term 'four point restraints' is indicative that four extremities have been restrained.

35. D
Cold packs are extremely therapeutic in the treatment of bruising, swelling and pain, however you should continually assess the patient's skin during their use and they should be limited to an application time not to exceed 20 minutes per treatment. The skin should then be reassessed and proper documentation performed.

36. A
For a minor injury, you should not see these symptoms. Blue-black tissue, intense pain and extremely cool skin could indicate a blood clot or more serious tissue damage than was originally thought. You should report your findings to the proper authority.

37. C
Always double-check your vital signs to make certain there is a valid problem.

38. C
While the thermometer is registering John's temperature, it is a good time to count his respirations. This is an example of good time management.

39. D
The respiratory assessment should ALWAYS include the number of respirations, the quality of them and accompanying breath sounds.

40. D
A child of this age could have her b/p assessed on any of the above-mentioned areas using a child's cuff.

41. A
Within the 5 hours you have been on duty, given that you are to assess his vital signs every 4 hours, you should have documented them twice.

42. B
When noting vital signs you must give as much information as you have been able to obtain. This should include the count, quality, and anything abnormal.

43. D
An oral thermometer is never used to take a rectal temperature. Gloves, lubricant and a rectal thermometer are the appropriate implements utilized during this phase of vital signs.

44. A
Anger is one of the stages of grief and Joyce has just experienced the loss of a loved one.

45. B
You must be willing to talk to her about death. At some point, this is something that any patient who experiences a loss will do.

46. A
Setting boundaries for sexual conduct in the workplace is important.

47. A
You should always document harassment of any kind as well as your response. It is your protection. Remember, if you don't document, it NEVER happened.

48. D
Joyce is exhibiting symptoms of withdrawal and silence. She is not talking, actively grieving, or crying.

49. B
Paraphrasing is restating something that a patient has said, usually in fewer words and with emphasis on the main points of their statement.

50. B
Facial expression, posture and tone of voice are elements of nonverbal communication.

51. D
Nonverbal communications can emphasize or contradict verbal messages is the only statement that is true.

52. C
Nodding provides encourages the patient to continue talking without indicating agreement or disagreement.

53. A
Using phrases that address a person's feelings, such as "You must be worried about your headaches," demonstrates empathy.

54. D
Always address older patients Miss, Mrs., or Mr., followed by their last name. Addressing older patients by their first name may offend.

55. A
When interviewing a patient with a hearing loss, remember to speak slowly and look directly at the patient.

56. D
In a health care facility, such as a hospital, nursing home, or assisted living, an incident report or accident report is a form that is filled out in order to record details of an unusual event that occurs at the facility, such as an injury to a patient. The purpose of the incident report is to document the exact details of the occurrence while they are fresh in the minds of those who witnessed the event. This information may be useful in the future when dealing with liability issues stemming from the incident.
Generally, according to health care guidelines, the report must be filled out as soon as possible following the incident (but after the situation has been stabilized). This way, the details written in the report are as accurate as possible.

Most incident reports that are written involve accidents with patients, such as patient falls. But most facilities will also document an incident in which a staff member or visitor is injured.

In the event that an incident involves a patient, the patient will often be monitored for a period of time following the incident (for it may happen again), which may include taking vital signs regularly. 3

57. C
Using neutral remarks such as, "I see" and "I hear what you're saying" indicates understanding to the patient.

58. A
If a patient refuses to make eye contact, you may find that they are from a culture that considers direct eye contact rude.

59. A
Speak slowly and carefully. Raising your voice will not help.

60. C
A geriatrician's practice is limited to persons over the age of 65 is false. Geriatrics is a sub-specialty of internal medicine and family medicine that focuses on health care of elderly people. It aims to promote health by preventing and treating diseases and disabilities in older adults. There is no set age at which patients may be under the care of a geriatrician, or physician who specializes in the care of elderly people. Rather, this decision is determined by the individual patient's needs, and the availability of a specialist.[4]

How to Prepare for a Test

MOST STUDENTS HIDE THEIR HEADS AND PROCRASTINATE WHEN FACED WITH PREPARING FOR AN EXAMINATION, HOPING THAT SOMEHOW THEY WILL BE SPARED THE AGONY OF TAKING THAT TEST, ESPECIALLY IF IT IS A BIG ONE THAT THEIR FUTURES RELY ON. Avoiding the all-important test is what many students do best and unfortunately, they suffer the consequences because of their lack of preparation.

Test preparation requires strategy. It also requires a dedication to getting the job done. It is the perfect training ground for anyone planning a professional life. In addition to having a number of reliable strategies, the wise student also has a clear goal in mind and knows how to accomplish it. These tried and true concepts have worked well and will make your test preparation easier.

The Study Approach.

Take responsibility for your own test preparation.

It is a common- but big - mistake to link your studying to someone else's. Study partners are great, but only if they are reliable. It is your job to be prepared for the test, even if a study partner fails you. Do not allow others to distract you from your goals.

Prioritize the time available to study.

When do you learn best, early in the day or in the dark of night? Does your mind absorb and retain information most efficiently in small blocks of time, or do you require long stretches to get the most done? It is important to figure out the best blocks of time available to you when you can be the most productive. Try to consolidate activities to allow for longer periods of study time.

Find a quiet place where you will not be disturbed.

Do not try to squeeze in quality study time in any old location. Find someplace peaceful and with a minimum of distractions, such as the library, a park or even the laundry room. Good lighting is essential and you need to have comfortable seating and a desk surface large enough to hold your materials. It is probably not a great idea to study in your bedroom. You might be distracted by clothes on the floor, a book you have been planning to read, the telephone or something else. Besides, in the middle of studying, that bed will start to look very comfortable. Whatever you do, avoid using the bed as a place to study since you might fall asleep as a way of avoiding your work! That is the last thing you should be doing during study time.

The exception is flashcards. By far the most productive study time is sitting down and studying and studying only. However, with flashcards you can carry them with you and make use of odd moments, like standing in line or waiting for the bus. This isn't as productive, but it really helps and is definitely worth doing.

Determine what you need in order to study.

Gather together your books, your notes, your laptop and any other materials needed to focus on your study for this exam. Ensure you have everything you need so you don't waste time. Remember paper, pencils and erasers, sticky notes, bottled water and a snack. Keep your phone with you in case you need it to find out essential information, but keep it turned off so others can't distract you.

Have a positive attitude.

It is essential that you approach your studies for the test with an attitude that says you will pass it. And pass it with flying colors! This is one of the most important keys to successful study strategy. Believing that you are capable actually helps you to become capable.

Study >> Practice >> Succeed!   Complete Test Preparation

The Strategy of Studying

Make materials easy to review and access.

Consolidate materials to help keep your study area clutter free. If you have a laptop and a means of getting on line, you do not need a dictionary and thesaurus as well since those things are easily accessible via the internet. Go through written notes and consolidate those, as well. Have everything you need, but do not weigh yourself down with duplicates.

Review class notes.

Stay on top of class notes and assignments by reviewing them frequently. Re-writing notes can be a terrific study trick, as it helps lock in information. Pay special attention to any comments that have been made by the teacher. If a study guide has been made available as part of the class materials, use it! It will be a valuable tool to use for studying.

Estimate how much time you will need.

If you are concerned about the amount of time you have available it is a good idea to set up a schedule so that you do not get bogged down on one section and end up without enough time left to study other things. Remember to schedule break time, and use that time for a little exercise or other stress reducing techniques.

Test yourself to determine your weaknesses.

Look online for additional assessment and evaluation tools available for a particular subject. Once you have determined areas of concern, you will be able to focus on studying the information they contain and just brush up on the other areas of the exam.

Mental Prep – How to Psych Yourself Up for a Test

Because tests contribute mightily to your final class grade or to whether you are accepted into a program, it is understandable that taking tests can create a great deal of anxiety for many students. Even students who know they have learned all of the required material find their minds going blank as they stare at the words in the questions. One of the easiest ways to overcome that anxiety is to prepare mentally for the test. Mentally preparing for an exam is really not difficult. There are simple techniques that any student can learn to increase their chances of earning a great score on the day of the test.

Do not procrastinate.

Study the material for the test when it becomes available, and continue to review the material up until the test day. By waiting until the last minute and trying to cram for the test the night before, you actually increase the amount of anxiety you feel. This leads to an increase in negative self-talk. Telling yourself "I can't learn this. I am going to fail" is a pretty sure indication that you are right. At best, your performance on the test will not be as strong if you have procrastinated instead of studying.

Positive self-talk.

Positive self-talk serves both to drown out negative self-talk and to increase your confidence in your abilities. Whenever you begin feeling overwhelmed or anxious about the test, remind yourself that you have studied enough, you know the material and that you will pass the test. Use only positive words. Both negative and positive self-talk are really just your fantasy, so why not choose to be a winner?

Study >> Practice >> Succeed!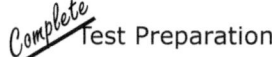

Do not compare yourself to anyone else.

Do not compare yourself to other students, or your performance to theirs. Instead, focus on your own strengths and weaknesses and prepare accordingly. Regardless of how others perform, your performance is the only one that matters to your grade. Comparing yourself to others increases your anxiety and your level of negative self-talk before the test.

Visualize.

Make a mental image of yourself taking the test. You know the answers and feel relaxed. Visualize doing well on the test and having no problems with the material. Visualizations can increase your confidence and decrease the anxiety you might otherwise feel before the test. Instead of thinking of this as a test, see it as an opportunity to demonstrate what you have learned!

Avoid negativity.

Worry is contagious and viral - once it gets started it builds on itself. Cut it off before it gets to be a problem. Even if you are relaxed and confident, being around anxious, worried classmates might cause you to start feeling anxious. Before the test, tune out the fears of classmates. Feeling anxious and worried before an exam is normal, and every student experiences those feelings at some point. But you cannot allow these feelings to interfere with your ability to perform well. Practicing mental preparation techniques and remembering that the test is not the only measure of your academic performance will ease your anxiety and ensure that you perform at your best.

How to Take a Test

EVERYONE KNOWS THAT TAKING AN EXAM IS STRESSFUL, BUT IT DOES NOT HAVE TO BE THAT BAD! There are a few simple things that you can do to increase your score on any type of test. Take a look at these tips and consider how you can incorporate them into your study time.

How to Take a Test - The Basics.

Some tests are designed to assess your ability to quickly grab the necessary information; this type of exam makes speed a priority. Others are more concerned with your depth of knowledge, and how accurate it is. When you receive a test, look it over to determine whether the test is for speed or accuracy. If the test is for speed, like many standardized tests, your strategy is clear; answer as many questions as quickly as possible.

Watch out, though! There are a few tests that are designed to determine how fully and accurately you can answer the questions. Guessing on this type of test is a big mistake, because the teacher expects any student with an average grade to be able to complete the test in the time given. Racing through the test and making guesses that prove to be incorrect will cost you big time!

Every little bit helps.

If you are permitted calculators, or other materials, make sure you bring them, even if you do not think you will need them. Use everything at your disposal to increase your score.

Make time your friend.

Budget your time from the moment your pencil hits the page until you are finished with the exam, and stick to it! Virtually all standardized tests have a time limit for each section. The amount of time you are permitted for each portion of the test will almost certainly be included in the instructions or printed at the top of the page. If for some reason it is not immediately visible, rather than wasting your time hunting for it you can use the points or percentage of the score as a proxy to make an educated guess regarding the time limit.

Use the allotted time for each section and then move on to the next section whether you have completed the first section or not. Stick with the instructions and you will be able to answer the majority of the questions in each section.

With speed tests you may not be able to complete the entire test. Rest assured that you are not really expected to! The goal of this type of examination is to determine how quickly you can reach into your brain and access a particular piece of information, which is one way of determining how well you know it. If you know a test you are taking is a speed test, you will know the strategies to use for the best results.

Read the directions carefully.

Spend a few minutes reading the directions carefully before starting each section. Studies show students who read the instructions get higher marks! If you just glance at them, you may misunderstand and could blow the whole thing. Very small changes in the wording of the instructions or the punctuation can change the meaning completely. Do not make assumptions. Just because the directions are written one way in one section does not mean they will be exactly the same in all sections. Focus your attention and read what the instructions actually say, not what you think they are saying.

Study >> Practice >> Succeed!

When reading the directions, underline the important parts. For example, if you are directed to circle the best answer, underline "circle" and "best". This flags the key concepts and will keep you focused.

If the exam is given with an answer booklet, copy the instructions to the top of the first page in the booklet. For complicated instructions, divide the directions into smaller steps and number each part.

Easy does it.

One smart way to tackle a test is to locate the easy questions and answer those first. This is a time-tested strategy that never fails, because it saves you a lot of unnecessary fretting. First, read the question and decide if you can answer it in less than a minute. If so, complete the question and go on to the next one. If not, skip it for now and continue on to the next question. By the time you have completed the first pass through this section of the exam, you will have answered a good number of questions. Not only does it boost your confidence, relieve anxiety and kick your memory up a notch, you will know exactly how many questions remain and can allot the rest of your time accordingly. Think of doing the easy questions first as a warm-up!

If you run out of time before you manage to tackle all the difficult questions, do not let it throw you. All that means is you have used your time in the most efficient way possible by answering as many questions correctly as you could. Missing a few points by not answering a question whose answer you do not know just means you spent that time answering one whose answer you did.

A word to the wise: Skipping questions for which you are drawing a complete blank is one thing, but we are not suggesting you skip every question you come across that you are not 100 % certain of. A good rule of thumb is to try to answer at least eight of every 10 questions the first time through.

Do not watch your watch.

At best, taking an important exam is an uncomfortable situation. If you are like most people, you might be tempted to subconsciously distract yourself from the task at hand. One of the most common ways to do so is by becoming obsessed with your watch or the wall clock. Do not watch your watch! Take it off and place it on the top corner of your desk, far enough away that you will not be tempted to look at it every two minutes. Better still, turn the watch face away from you. That way, every time you try to sneak a peek, you will be reminded to refocus your attention to the task at hand. Give yourself permission to check your watch or the wall clock after you complete each section. If you know yourself to be a bit of a slow-poke in other aspects of life, you can check your watch a bit more often. Even so, focus on answering the questions, not on how many minutes have elapsed since you last looked at it.

Divide and conquer.

What should you do when you come across a question that is so complicated you may not even be certain what is being asked? As we have suggested, the first time through the section you are best off skipping the question. But at some point, you will need to return to it and get it under control. The best way to handle questions that leave you feeling so anxious you can hardly think is by breaking them into manageable pieces. Solving smaller bits is always easier. For complicated questions, divide them into bite-sized pieces and solve these smaller sets separately. Once you understand what the reduced sections are really saying, it will be much easier to put them together and get a handle on the bigger question.

Reason your way through the toughest questions.

If you find that a question is so dense you can't figure out how to break it into smaller pieces, there are a few strategies that might help. First, read the question again and look for hints. Can you re-word the question in one or more different ways? This may give you clues. Look for words that can function as either verbs or nouns, and try to figure out from the sentence structure which it is in this case. Remember that many nouns in English have a number of different meanings. While some of those meanings might be related, in some cases they are completely distinct. If reading the sentence one way does not make sense, consider a different definition or meaning for a key word.

The truth is, it is not always necessary to understand a question to arrive at a correct answer! A trick that successful students understand is using Strategy 5, Elimination. In many cases, at least one answer is clearly wrong and can be crossed off of the list of possible correct answers. Next, look at the remaining answers and eliminate any that are only partially true. You may still have to flat-out guess from time to time, but using the process of elimination will help you make your way to the correct answer more often than not - even when you don't know what the question means!

Do not leave early.

Use all the time allotted to you, even if you can't wait to get out of the testing room. Instead, once you have finished, spend the remaining time reviewing your answers. Go back to those questions that were most difficult for you and review your response. Another good way to use this time is to return to multiple choice questions in which you filled in a bubble. Do a spot check, reviewing every fifth or sixth question to make sure your answer coincides with the bubble you filled in. This is a great way to catch yourself if you made a mistake, skipped a bubble and therefore put all your answers in the wrong bubbles!

Become a super sleuth and look for careless errors. Look for questions that have double negatives or other odd phrasing; they might be an attempt to throw you off. Careless errors on your part might be the result of skimming a question and missing a key word. Words such as "always", "never", "sometimes" , "rarely" and the like can give a strong indication of the answer the question is really seeking. Don't throw away points by being careless!

Just as you budgeted time at the beginning of the test to allow for easy and more difficult questions, be sure to budget sufficient time to review your answers. On essay questions and math questions where you are required to show your work, check your writing to make sure it is legible.

Math questions can be especially tricky. The best way to double check math questions is by figuring the answer using a different method, if possible.

Here is another terrific tip. It is likely that no matter how hard you try, you will have a handful of questions you just are not sure of. Keep them in mind as you read through the rest of the test. If you can't answer a question, looking back over the test to find a different question that addresses the same topic might give you clues.

We know that taking the test has been stressful and you can hardly wait to escape. Just keep in mind that leaving before you double-check as much as possible can be a quick trip to disaster. Taking a few extra minutes can make the difference between getting a bad grade and a great one. Besides, there will be lots of time to relax and celebrate after the test is turned in.

In the Test Room – What you MUST do!

If you are like the rest of the world, there is almost nothing you would rather avoid than taking a test. Unfortunately, that is not an option if you want to pass. Rather than suffer, consider a few attitude adjustments that might turn the experience from a horrible one to…well, an interesting one! Take a look at these tips. Simply changing how you perceive the experience can change the experience itself.

Get in the mood.

After weeks of studying, the big day has finally arrived. The worst thing you can do to yourself is arrive at the test site feeling frustrated, worried, and anxious. Keep a check on your emotional state. If your emotions are shaky before a test it can determine how well you do on the test. It is extremely important that you pump yourself up, believe in yourself, and use that confidence to get in the mood!

Don't fight reality.

Oftentimes, students resent tests, and with good reason. After all, many people do not test well, and they know the grade they end up with does not accurately reflect their true knowledge. It is easy to feel resentful because tests classify students and create categories that just don't seem fair. Face it: Students who are great at rote memorization and not that good at actually analyzing material often score higher than those who might be more creative thinkers and balk at simply memorizing cold, hard facts. It may not be fair, but there it is anyway. Conformity is an asset on tests, and creativity is often a liability. There is no point in wasting time or energy being upset about this reality. Your first step is to accept the reality and get used to it. You will get higher marks when you realize tests do count and that you must give them your best effort. Think about your future and the career that is easier to achieve if you have consistently earned high grades. Avoid negative energy and focus on anything that lifts your enthusiasm and increases your motivation.

Get there early enough to relax.

If you are wound up, tense, scared, anxious, or feeling rushed, it will cost you. Get to the exam room early and relax before you go in. This way, when the exam starts, you are comfortable and ready to apply yourself. Of course, you do not want to arrive so early that you are the only one there. That will not help you relax; it will only give you too much time to sit there, worry and get wound up all over again.

If you can, visit the room where you will be taking your exam a few days ahead of time. Having a visual image of the room can be surprisingly calming, because it takes away one of the big 'unknowns'. Not only that, but once you have visited, you know how to get there and will not be worried about getting lost. Furthermore, driving to the test site once lets you know how much time you need to allow for the trip. That means three potential stressors have been eliminated all at once.

Get it down on paper.

One of the advantages of arriving early is that it allows you time to recreate notes. If you spend a lot of time worrying about whether you will be able to remember information like names, dates, places, and mathematical formulas, there is a solution for that. Unless the exam you are taking allows you to use your books and notes, (and very few do) you will have to rely on memory. Arriving early gives to time to tap into your memory and jot down key pieces of information you know will be asked. Just make certain you are allowed to make notes once you are in the testing site; not all locations will permit it. Once you get your test, on a small piece of paper write down everything you are afraid you will forget. It will take a minute or two but by dumping your worries onto the page you have effectively eliminated a certain amount of anxiety and driven off the panic you feel.

Get comfortable in your chair.

Here is a clever technique that releases physical stress and helps you get comfortable, even relaxed in your body. You will tense and hold each of your muscles for just a few seconds. The trick is, you must tense them hard for the technique to work. You might want to practice this technique a few times at home; you do not want an unfamiliar technique to add to your stress just before a test, after all! Once you are at the test site, this exercise can always be done in the rest room or another quiet location.

Start with the muscles in your face then work down your body. Tense, squeeze and hold the muscles for a moment or two. Notice the feel of every muscle as you go down your body. Scowl to tense your forehead, pull in your chin to tense your neck. Squeeze your shoulders down to tense your back. Pull in your stomach all the way back to your ribs, make your lower back tight then stretch your fingers. Tense your leg muscles and calves then stretch your feet and your toes. You should be as stiff as a board throughout your entire body.

Now relax your muscles in reverse starting with your toes. Notice how all the muscles feel as you relax them one by one. Once you have released a muscle or set of muscles, allow them to remain relaxed as you proceed up your body. Focus on how you are feeling as all the tension leaves. Start breathing deeply when you get to your chest muscles. By the time you have found your chair, you will be so relaxed it will feel like bliss!

Fight distraction.

A lucky few are able to focus deeply when taking an important examination, but most people are easily distracted, probably because they would rather be anyplace else! There are a number of things you can do to protect yourself from distraction.

Stay away from windows. If you select a seat near a window you may end up gazing out at the landscape instead of paying attention to the work at hand. Furthermore, any sign of human activity, from a single individual walking by to a couple having an argument or exchanging a kiss will draw your attention away from your important work. What goes on outside should not be allowed to distract you.

Choose a seat away from the aisle so you do not become distracted by people who leave early. People who leave the exam room early are often the ones who fail. Do not compare your time to theirs.

Of course you love your friends; that's why they are your friends! In the test room, however, they should become complete strangers inside your mind. Forget they are there. The first step is to physically distance yourself from friends or classmates. That way, you will not be tempted to glance at them to see how they are doing, and there will be no chance of eye contact that could either distract you or even lead to an accusation of cheating. Furthermore, if they are feeling stressed because they did not spend the focused time studying that you did, their anxiety is less likely to permeate your hard-earned calm.

Of course, you will want to choose a seat where there is sufficient light. Nothing is worse than trying to take an important examination under flickering lights or dim bulbs.

Ask the instructor or exam proctor to close the door if there is a lot of noise outside. If the instructor or proctor is unable to do so, block out the noise as best you can. Do not let anything disturb you.

Make sure you have enough pencils, pens and whatever else you will need. Many entrance exams do not permit you to bring personal items such as candy bars into the testing room. If this is the case with the exam you are sitting for, be sure to eat a nutritionally balanced breakfast. Eat protein, complex carbohydrates and a little fat to keep you feeling full and to supercharge your energy. Nothing is worse than a sudden drop in blood sugar during an exam.

Do not allow yourself to become distracted by being too cold or hot. Regardless of the weather outside, carry a sweater, scarf or jacket in case the air conditioning at the test site is set too high, or the heat set too low. By the same token, dress in layers so that you are prepared for a range of temperatures.

Bring a watch so that you can keep track of time management. The danger here is many students become obsessed with how many minutes have passed since the last question. Instead of wearing the watch, remove it and place it in the far upper corner of the desk with the face turned away. That way, you cannot become distracted by repeatedly glancing at the time, but it is available if you need to know it.

Drinking a gallon of coffee or gulping a few energy drinks might seem like a great idea, but it is, in fact, a very bad one. Caffeine, pep pills or other artificial sources of energy are more likely to leave you feeling rushed and ragged. Your brain might be clicking along, all right, but chances are good it is not clicking along on the right track! Furthermore, drinking lots of coffee or energy drinks will mean frequent trips to the rest room. This will cut into the time you should be spending answering questions and is a distraction in itself, since each time you need to leave the room you lose focus. Pep pills will only make it harder for you to think straight when solving complicated problems on the exam.

At the same time, if anxiety is your problem try to find ways around using tranquilizers during test-taking time. Even medically prescribed anti-anxiety medication can make you less alert and even decrease your motivation. Being motivated is what you need to get you through an exam. If your anxiety is so bad that it threatens to interfere with your ability to take an exam, speak to your doctor and ask for documentation. Many testing sites will allow non-distracting test rooms, extended testing time and other accommodations as long as a doctor's note that explains the situation is made available.

Keep Breathing.

It might not make a lot of sense, but when people become anxious, tense, or scared, their breathing becomes shallow and, in some cases, they stop breathing all together! Pay attention to your emotions, and when you are feeling worried, focus on your breathing. Take a moment to remind yourself to breathe deeply and regularly. Drawing in steady, deep breaths energizes the body. When you continue to breathe deeply you will notice you exhale all the tension.

It is a smart idea to rehearse breathing at home. With continued practice of this relaxation technique, you will begin to know the muscles that tense up under pressure. Call these your "signal muscles." These are the ones that will speak to you first, begging you to relax. Take the time to listen to those muscles and do as they ask. With just a little breathing practice, you will get into the habit of checking yourself regularly and when you realize you are tense, relaxation will become second nature.

Avoid Anxiety Prior to a Test

Manage your time effectively.

This is a key to your success! You need blocks of uninterrupted time to study all the pertinent material. Creating and maintaining a schedule will help keep you on track, and will remind family members and friends that you are not available. Under no circumstances should you change your blocks of study time to accommodate someone else, or cancel a study session in order to do something more fun. Do not interfere with your study time for any reason!

Relax.

Use whatever works best for you to relieve stress. Some folks like a good, calming stretch with yoga, others find expressing themselves through journaling to be useful. Some hit the floor for a series of crunches or planks, and still others take a slow stroll around the garden. Integrate a little relaxation time into your schedule, and treat that time, too, as sacred.

Eat healthy.

Instead of reaching for the chips and chocolate, fresh fruits and vegetables are not only yummy but offer nutritional benefits that help to relieve stress. Some foods accelerate stress instead of reducing it and should be avoided. Foods that add to higher anxiety include artificial sweeteners, candy and other sugary foods, carbonated sodas, chips, chocolate, eggs, fried foods, junk foods, processed foods, red meat, and other foods containing preservatives or heavy spices. Instead, eat a bowl of berries and some yogurt!

Get plenty of ZZZZZZZs.

Do not cram or try to do an all-nighter. If you created a study schedule at the beginning, and if you have stuck with that schedule, have confidence! Staying up too late trying to cram in last-minute bits of information is going to leave you exhausted the next day. Besides, whatever new information you cram in will only displace all the important ideas you've spent weeks learning. Remember: You need to be alert and fully functional the day of the exam

Eat a healthy meal before the exam.

Whatever you do - do not go into the test room hungry! Eat a meal that is rich in protein and complex carbohydrates before the test. Avoid sugary foods; they will pump you up initially, but you might crash hard part way through the exam. While you do not want to consume a lot of unhealthy fat, you do need a little of the healthy stuff such as flaxseed or olive oil on a salad. Avoid fried foods; they tend to make you sleepy.

Have confidence in yourself!

Everyone experiences some anxiety when taking a test, but exhibiting a positive attitude banishes anxiety and fills you with the knowledge you really do know what you need to know. This is your opportunity to show how well prepared you are. Go for it!

Be sure to take everything you need.

Depending on the exam, you may be allowed to have a pen or pencil, calculator, dictionary or scratch paper with you.

Study >> Practice >> Succeed!   Complete Test Preparation

Have these gathered together along with your entrance paperwork and identification so that you are sure you have everything that is needed.

Do not chitchat with friends.

Let your friends know ahead of time that it is not anything personal, but you are going to ignore them in the test room! You need to find a seat away from doors and windows, one that has good lighting, and get comfortable. If other students are worried their anxiety could be detrimental to you; of course, you do not have to tell your friends that. If you are afraid they will be offended, tell them you are protecting them from your anxiety!

Common Test-Taking Mistakes

Taking a test is not much fun at best. When you take a test and make a stupid mistake that negatively affects your grade, it is natural to be very upset, especially when it is something that could have been easily avoided. So what are some of the common mistakes that are made on tests?

Do not fail to put your name on the test.

How could you possibly forget to put your name on a test? You would be amazed at how often that happens. Very often, tests without names are thrown out immediately, resulting in a failing grade.

Not following directions.

Directions are carefully worded. If you skim directions, it is very easy to miss key words or misinterpret what is being said. Nothing is worse than failing an examination simply because you could not be bothered with reading the instructions!

Marking The Wrong Multiple Choice Answer.

It is important to work at a steady pace, but that does not mean bolting through the questions. Be sure the answer you are marking is the one you mean to. If the bubble you need to fill in or the answer you need to circle is 'C', do not allow yourself to get distracted and select 'B' instead.

Answering A Question Twice.

Some multiple choice test questions have two very similar answers. If you are in too much of a hurry, you might select them both. Remember that only one answer is correct, so if you choose more than one, you have automatically failed that question.

Mishandling A Difficult Question.

We recommend skipping difficult questions and returning to them later, but beware! First of all, be certain that you do return to the question. Circling the entire passage or placing a large question mark beside it will help you spot it when you are reviewing your test. Secondly, if you are not careful to actually skip the question, you can mess yourself up badly. Imagine that a question is too difficult and you decide to save it for later. You read the next question, which you know the answer to, and you fill in that answer. You continue on to the end of the test then return to the difficult question only to discover you didn't actually skip it! Instead, you inserted the answer to the following question in the spot reserved for the harder one, thus throwing off the remainder of your test!

Study >> Practice >> Succeed!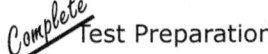

Incorrectly Transferring An Answer From Scratch Paper.

This can happen easily if you are trying to hurry! Double check any answer you have figured out on scratch paper, and make sure what you have written on the test itself is an exact match!

Don't Ignoring The Clock, And Don't Marry It, Either.

In a timed examination many students lose track of the time and end up without sufficient time to complete the test. Remember to pace yourself! At the same time, though, do not allow yourself to become obsessed with how much time has elapsed, either.

Thinking Too Much.

Oftentimes, your first thought is your best thought. If you worry yourself into insecurity, your self-doubts can trick you into choosing an incorrect answer when your first impulse was the right one!

Be Prepared.

Running out of ink and not having an extra pen or pencil is not an excuse for failing an exam! Have everything you need, and have extras. Bring tissue, an extra erasure, several sharpened pencils, batteries for electronic devices, and anything else you might need.

Conclusion

CONGRATULATIONS! You have made it this far because you have applied yourself diligently to practicing for the exam and no doubt improved your potential score considerably! Getting into a good school is a huge step in a journey that might be challenging at times but will be many times more rewarding and fulfilling. That is why being prepared is so important.

Study then Practice and then Succeed!

Good Luck!

Thanks!

If you enjoyed this book and would like to order additional copies for yourself or for friends, please check with your local bookstore, favourite online bookseller or visit www.test-preparation.ca and place your order directly with the publisher.

Feedback to the publisher may be sent by email to feed-back@test-preparation.ca

Customizing and White Label Service

Have your logo and school name on the front cover in a special edition produced for your school or institution. Visit http://test-preparation.ca/customization.html or please contact us for details at sales@test-preparation.ca

Study >> Practice >> Succeed!

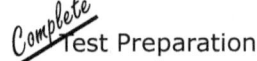

NOTES

Text where noted below is used under the Creative Commons Attribution-ShareAlike 3.0 License

http://en.wikipedia.org/wiki/Wikipedia:Text_of_Creative_Commons_Attribution-ShareAlike_3.0_Unported_License

[1] Influenza. In *Wikipedia*. Retrieved January 22, 2012 from http://en.wikipedia.org/wiki/Influenza.
[2] Advance Directive. In *Wikipedia*. Retrieved January 22, 2012 from http://en.wikipedia.org/wiki/Advance_directive.
[3] Incident Report. In *Wikipedia*. Retrieved January 22, 2012 from http://en.wikipedia.org/wiki/Incident_report
[4] Geriatrician. In *Wikipedia*. Retrieved January 22, 2012 from http://en.wikipedia.org/wiki/Geriatrician

www.ingramcontent.com/pod-product-compliance
Lightning Source LLC
Chambersburg PA
CBHW061515180526
45171CB00001B/189